The *Book* *of*
Slimming
Tips

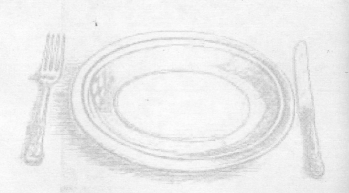

To David

The Little Book
of
Slimming Tips

J U D Y   C I T R O N

the **D**ietCoach

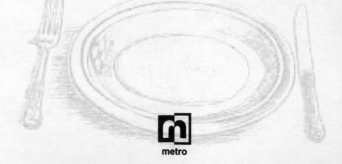

n

metro

First published in Great Britain in 2000
by Metro Books (an imprint of Metro Publishing
Limited), 19 Gerrard Street, London W1V 7LA

British Library Cataloguing in Publication Data.
A CIP record of this book is available on request
from the British Library.

ISBN 1 900512 94 7

10 9 8 7 6 5 4 3 2 1

Printed in Great Britain by
Omnia Books Limited, Glasgow

Introduction

I used to be overweight. I struggled for years, trying every diet on the shelves. Often I lost weight but I always put it back on and I saw this as my own fault – my lack of will-power – rather than the failure of the diets themselves. It wasn't until I stopped dieting that I lost weight and kept it off. Now I help others do the same.

If you've bought this book then it means that you're still hopeful that you can lose weight and keep that weight off. Like so many others who are struggling with their weight, you say to yourself that this time you'll do better.

But is it actually you who needs to do better? We're too ready to say that we – and our lack of will-power – are to blame. I have written this book because I want you to know that it's not your fault. It's the fault of the many diets out there. They display a frightening similarity and a total disregard of the trend: that more people than ever are on a diet yet more people than ever are overweight.

In this little book, therefore, I would like to appeal to you to try something different. Just as I did, have the courage to say, 'If I've tried so many diets and every time the weight goes back on, then maybe it's not me at fault but the diets.' It's time for a change.

Here's the biggest change. In these pages you'll find scant reference to specific foods and there are certainly no recipes. My objective is to change your focus away from the 'what' of eating. Conventional diets are quick to tell you to avoid this and keep off that; add up your calories and count your fat units. But that isn't the way forward. That's the way to increasing your obsession with food; it's the way to deprivation; it's the way back to bingeing and to yo-yo dieting and unhappiness. It's not the way to permanent weight loss.

I'd like to persuade you that the traditional emphasis on what you eat, is far less important than the why, where, when and how of eating.

You already know what to eat. You're probably a walking calorie counter. Journey with me to ask different questions and you'll get better answers.

Motivational gurus have discovered that if you want to achieve success you should ask a successful person how they function. In the same way, if we want to lose weight permanently we have to try and understand the behaviour of slim people. Ask a naturally slim person why they eat and you will receive one simple answer: they eat because they're hungry. They are in touch with their natural appetite.

Ask yourself why you eat and, if you're honest, you'll probably reply that you eat because you're depressed; because you're angry; because you're tired; because you're bored or because eating is an acceptable way to take a break or to socialize.

Unfortunately, I can't lift your depression or your anger directly, but I can remind you that nor can food. It's a destructive, vicious circle. You eat because you feel bad and then you feel worse because you ate. It probably sounds very familiar to you, but you can break that cycle, and I hope that the tips in these pages will help you do that. I hope they will help you rekindle your natural appetite. You can relearn how to eat to live and not live to eat.

In the past I always looked for a quick fix, but those crash diets didn't have any effect on my long-term habits. They just made me confused and angry with myself. I had to accept that speed is not of the essence. Habits of a lifetime can't be overturned in a week or even a month. Once I decided that changes had to be for life, I began to make steady and irreversible progress and so do my clients.

I hope that this book will give you a new starting point. Some of the tips suggest things to do, while others suggest a new way of thinking. Open this book and choose, say, five tips. Promise yourself that you'll observe them faithfully for a week. Then next week choose another set. Gradually you will build up a new way of life that will take your weight off and keep it off for good. You will experience weight off your body and a great weight off your mind.

Learn from the past

Take a piece of paper and write down every single diet you remember going on. Then write down what happened at the end of each one and what you thought of it. If you've tried any diet more than once, list it for every time you did it. How long is the list? Are you still overweight? There's only one conclusion you can draw: diets don't work. Use this book instead.

Only eat when you're physically hungry

If you don't know if you're hungry,
then you aren't. Drink some water and
do something else for ten minutes,
then you'll know for sure.

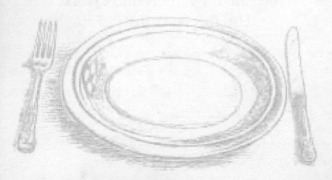

What's eating you?

If you want to eat when you're not physically hungry then work out what's eating you. What feelings are you burying with that mound of food. For example, you may conclude that you're lonely. One little step now may be to force yourself to phone someone you haven't spoken to for a long time.

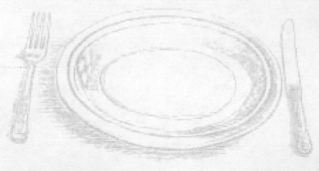

Eat more slowly and then slower still

If you eat slowly you'll savour your food and really appreciate it. Slow eating will also allow you to take smaller portions, no seconds and still be the last to finish. If your food gets cold because you are eating more slowly, put it in the microwave.

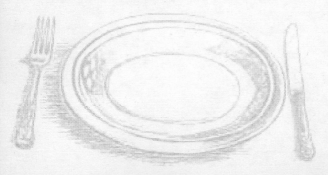

Learn to love food

Become a gourmet so you only eat food that you love and never eat food that isn't worth the calories.

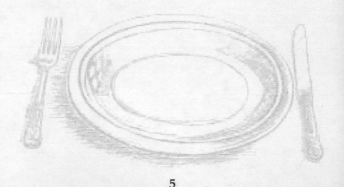

Never eat standing up

If you follow this rule and no other, you could probably lose half a pound a week until you reach your goal weight – and you'd stay there.

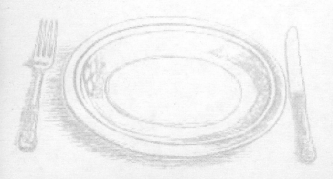

Think about where the food will sit itself

If you feel like eating but you're not physically hungry, ask yourself where on your body that food will settle. Imagine it on your hips or round your waist or wherever you least want it.

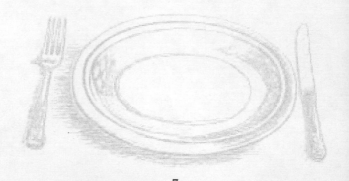

Become
a fidget

People who fidget burn more calories.
Move your feet round in circles; clench
then relax your fists; rub your hands
together; bounce your knees up and down
(but only when no one's looking).

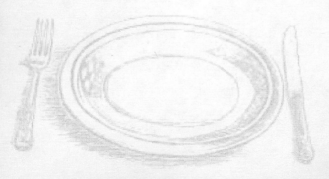

Don't feel like exercise? Do it anyway

Do you always feel like brushing your teeth? No – but you do it anyway. Make exercise exactly the same. Once you get past the first five minutes, enthusiasm will take over.

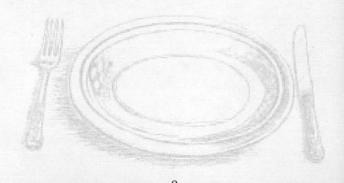

Don't wait for a crisis. An imaginary one will work too

Only one thing is certain if you are overweight; that sooner or later you will have a crisis. It may be that you can't find clothes to fit or your doctor gives you a health warning. Why wait for that crisis? Imagine it now and take action before it's a reality.

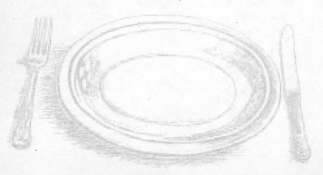

Do you dream
of becoming slim
and fit?

Dream on and it will become a reality.
This is one of the few dreams that
is completely in your hands to make
come true.

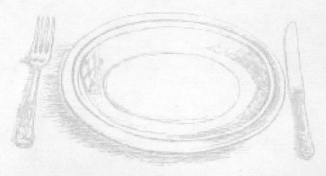

The bin is not a sin; it's your waist that is a waste

Of course you shouldn't cook more food than you can eat or take on your plate more than you need but, if you do, eating it is far worse than throwing it away. It won't help the world food shortage either way.

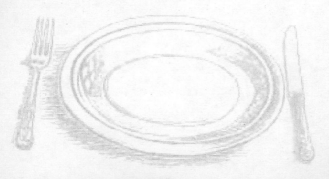

Never let your
food be boring

Each week choose something new in the
supermarket or local specialist food shop.
Pick an exotic fruit or a vegetable you've
never cooked before. Buy a new packet of
beans, or pulses. Borrow or buy a new
cookery book and get inspiration.

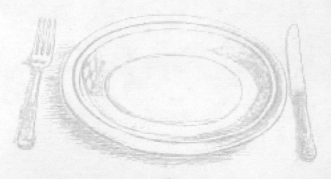

Never pick at the left-overs

When you've finished your meal and you're not hungry anymore, keep your hands out of the dishes. Imagine that you have gloves on and they're covered in mud.

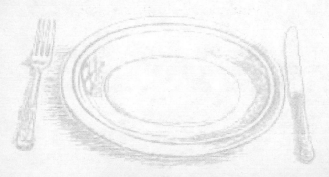

Never taste food while you're cooking

This one is particularly difficult for the real cooks among us, but for ordinary mortals, just follow the recipe and have faith. Tasting is only an excuse for some extra calories. If you've already put too much salt and pepper in, it's too late so why bother to taste? If there's too little, you can add it at the table.

Never go shopping when you're hungry

This is an old one, but worth repeating. You'll only buy your old favourites, your 'trigger' foods that may set you off into binge mode and everything unhealthy. If you're not hungry when you shop, you're more likely to choose healthy foods.

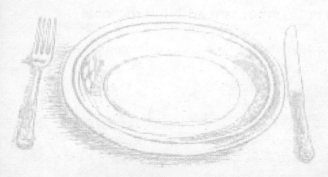

Drink water and then more water

Water is good for you. It keeps your bowels working, cleanses your system and enables you to postpone eating when you're not really hungry enough yet.

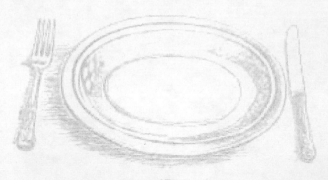

Imagine you're eating in front of a mirror

This little trick will help you eat more slowly. Just imagine what you look like when you're stuffing it in.

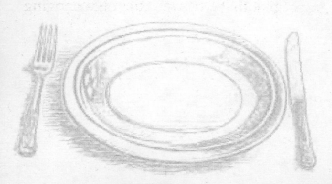

Make lists:
write down all the
disadvantages to
you of being
overweight

Start with some obvious ones like being
unhealthy and feeling uncomfortable. You
should be able to list up to 20 things. Now
imagine that list larger than life hanging
on every wall.

Make lists: write down all the advantages to you of being slim

The obvious ones are that you'll have more confidence, wear fashionable clothes and be healthier. Add your own personal dreams. Now imagine having achieved all of these. Make large images for yourself and see them in your mind's eye often.

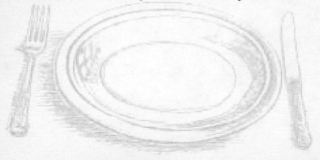

Whose life is it anyway?

You decide now, once and for all.
Weight loss is in your hands.
Are you going to let food boss you
around? You've got more strength
than that.

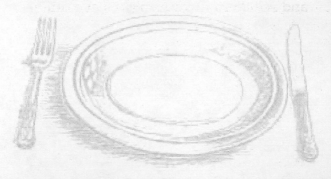

The buck stops with you

Do you blame your mother for your size?
Do you blame the media?
They may indeed be to blame but it's
only you who reaches out for the food.
No one is forcing you.

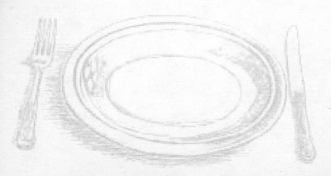

Don't generalize

You come to believe the generalizations. Do you ever say, 'I've never had any self-control'? Surely that's not true. Think of a time when you were really tempted – with food or anything else – but resisted. Never say 'never'.

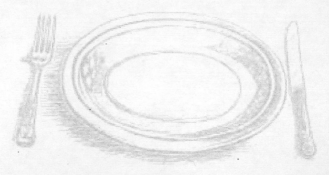

Don't make excuses

They don't convince anyone except you.
'I'd paid for it, so it was a waste not to eat
it.' 'It wouldn't have been fair to let my
friend eat alone.' You're not fooling
anyone. Accept that you slipped up and
cope better next time. Your hips don't
recognize excuses.

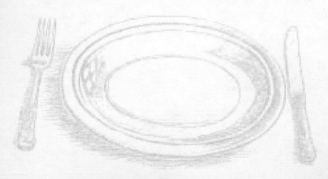

Choose two starters instead of a starter and a main course

In restaurants, main courses are often very large – more than you need to feel satisfied. If you're not very good at leaving food on your plate, choose two first courses. They're usually small and often delicious.

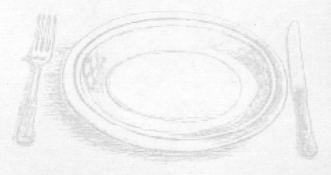

Put binges behind you – get back on course immediately

So you did carry on eating beyond being satisfied. No big deal. If you wait until you're hungry to eat next time, you'll be fine.

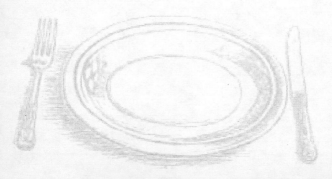

Put binges behind you – learn how not to do it next time

Try to work out what made you overeat.
If circumstances are the same again,
what could you do differently?

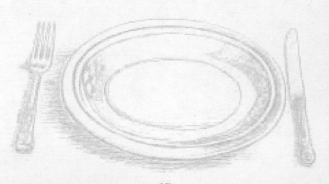

Talk to yourself firmly

When old habits rear their voices, stamp
on them. When you're about to give in to
a craving, tell yourself: 'Remember,
I don't do that anymore.' You will find
yourself obeying.

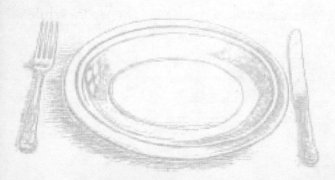

No time for exercise? Learn to do two things at once

You can certainly exercise while you watch television. You can exercise while you read the newspaper. You can exercise while you play with your children. You can exercise while you learn a language on cassette. What else can you do while you exercise?

Success breeds success

You resisted a second helping yesterday?
Re-live that experience vividly and feel a
glow of satisfaction. If you did it once,
you can do it again. What other successes
have you had? Build big pictures of them
in your mind.

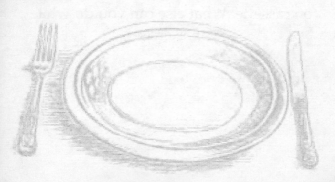

Develop the art of conversation

If you're eating in company, focus on the people. Make a conscious effort to be good company. Learn the art of asking questions and listening to the answers. You will eat more slowly and care less about the food.

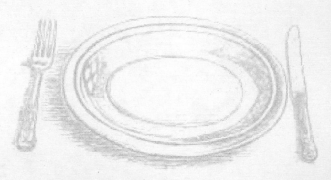

Learn the art of taking tiny bites

Slow eating is an essential art if you are to lose weight and keep it off permanently. See how long you can stretch out one biscuit. What about an apple? Cut it into tiny pieces and don't put a piece into your mouth until you've finished the one before it.

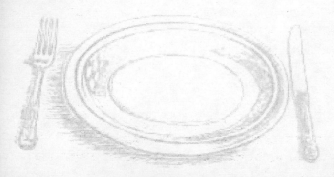

Put your knife and fork down between every bite

Sounds laborious but it works to slow you down so you'll never need a second helping. Imagine your fork attached to your plate with elastic. See the elastic pulling the fork back to your plate after each mouthful. Try it and then do it every time you eat.

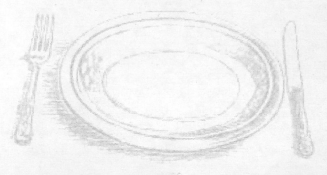

When a craving looms very large, go and brush your teeth

You know you're not physically hungry but that craving is about to get the better of you. Go and brush your teeth. It works wonders. The craving will have passed and you won't feel like eating.

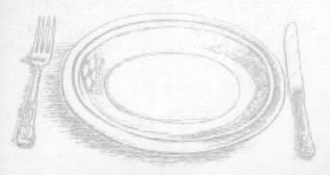

If weight loss is very slow, remember it's not a race, it's for life

You may feel as though you're doing everything right yet you've stopped losing weight. Stop looking at the scales and relax. What are the options? Slim or overweight. Which have you chosen? The decision is made – it doesn't matter if it takes a week more or a week less. It's for life, so just plod on.

Make lists of diversionary activities – and do them

If you sometimes eat because you're bored, make a list of even the most unlikely things to do. Go for a walk, stick photos in an album, clear out a cupboard, dance to some loud music. Get the idea? Now get the kit if you need any and do something from that list next time you're bored.

Start planning something new and exciting in your life

If you sometimes eat because you're bored, perhaps you need some new stimulation, a new goal or sense of achievement. What could you initiate? A new hobby? Learn a new skill? A new language? Find a new job? Meet new people? Take the first little step now.

Get those feelings down on paper

Do you eat when you feel low? Many of us eat to drown our sorrows. It's best to try and let them out instead of burying them under a mound of food. If there's no one to talk to then write your feelings down. If there's a particular person who is getting you down, write them a letter even if you never post it.

Ask yourself what you are avoiding

If you eat to procrastinate, find out why. Just another coffee and biscuit before you make that dreaded phone call? Ask yourself why you don't want to phone. Then ask why again. Go on questioning every answer you give. Eventually, you'll uncover something deep and decide what to do about it.

Release
that anger

If you eat when you're angry, run a
conversation in your head between you
and the person who has made you angry,
then go and have that conversation calmly
without anger. If you can't trust yourself
to do that, let off steam with some
physical activity. Punch a cushion; go for a
fast walk; run up and down stairs.

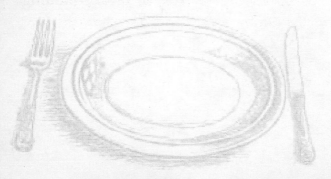

Learn relaxation techniques

If you eat when you're tense, learn to relax. Meditation is excellent; the next best thing is learning to breathe deeply. Not only will it divert you from eating when you're tense, it will also help you get to sleep at night and enhance your energy level. You don't have to wait until you're sitting comfortably either. You can breathe deeply while waiting for buses, queuing in the supermarket and so on.

Break the pattern

If you always eat popcorn at the cinema, choose an alternative and clutch it tightly. Clutch a hot cup of coffee or some diet coke. Decide not to have popcorn. Permitting yourself to have just a little probably won't work – like peanuts, popcorn is very 'moreish'. Sit at the end of the row and tell your friends not to pass the popcorn up to your end.

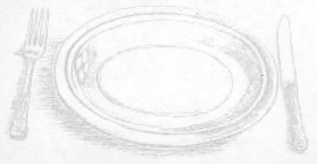

Occupy
your hands

If you always eat when you watch television, find something else to do with your hands. Try cat's cradle, knitting or using a stress ball. You might try doodling. Alternatively, put an exercise bicycle in front of the television and get on it. You're unlikely to eat while you're pedalling.

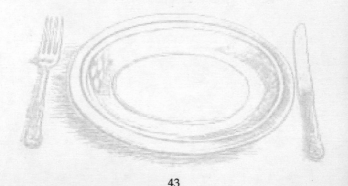

If dieting is getting you down, then lift someone else up

Dieting is slow, boring and best left on automatic pilot. But if it's getting you down because progress is slow, doing a good deed for someone else will give you an enormous lift. It will have the added benefit of giving a boost to the other person too.

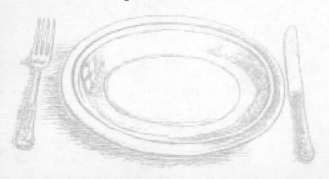

No food is forbidden

One of the reasons why diets don't work is because you put yourself through periods of great deprivation, then you get angry and eventually give in and go berserk. If you allow all foods to be eaten in moderate portions and always remember you can have more tomorrow, the 'forbidden' foods will eventually lose their appeal.

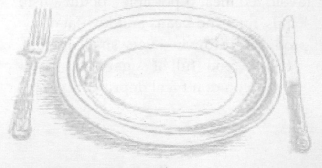

Learn about healthy, balanced nutrition

The basics of a balanced diet are simple. One third of your daily food (thinking about the room it takes on the plate) should be fruit and vegetables, one third should be potatoes, cereals, breads (wholegrain please), and the other third should be made up of protein foods (avoid red meat if possible), poultry, fish, lentils, nuts and beans and low-fat dairy products. Throw in a very small amount of 'junk' food (full of sugar and fat) so you don't feel deprived.

Slow but sure is the only route to permanent weight loss

Consider climbing a mountain. You can go up an almost sheer cliff but you're likely to slip down faster than you clambered up. You'll be out of breath and scared when you look back at the drop. But if you aim toward the summit along gentle slopes, you're not only sure to make it, but can also enjoy the view along the way.

Exercise doesn't have to be expensive

Fast walking must be one of the best and most inexpensive forms of exercise. A good pair of trainers helps, otherwise it's free. Then there's second-hand equipment (often advertised virtually unused in local newspapers). Find a bargain and make sure you're not the one trying to sell it next time round.

Exercise doesn't have to be formal

You can walk to work or walk the last few bus stops or the last station. You can park a few blocks away from home. You can walk up the escalator or stairs. Even being on the 22nd floor is no excuse. You can walk up the last few floors.

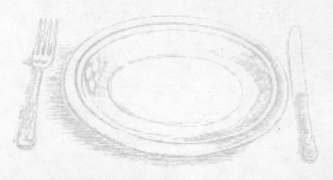

Exercise can be enjoyable (and if it's not, do it anyway)

Maybe you like competitive sports, or maybe not. Maybe you like it indoors or maybe outdoors. There is such a wide variety that there's no excuse for not finding something that you like.

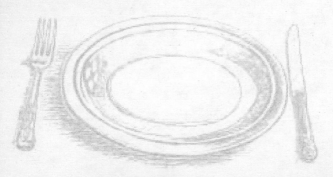

Exercise doesn't have to be boring

You can devise a different programme for every day of the week: indoor, outdoor, aerobic, strength, team or individual. You can exercise with a friend or colleague. You can get a group of people together and swap your equipment to ring the changes. You can buy second-hand equipment to widen your repertoire.

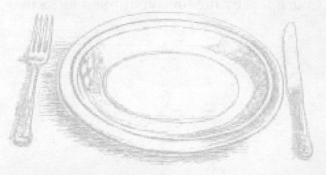

It takes your brain twenty minutes to notice that you've eaten

It's not your stomach that tells you that you've eaten enough, it's your brain. It takes your brain at least twenty minutes to get the message. So if you slow down in that twenty minutes you'll have eaten much less by the time your brain kicks in.

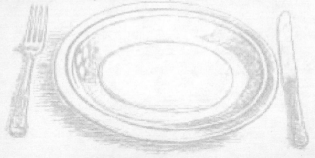

Never
'go on a diet'
again

Just look at the first three letters of 'diet'.
Yes, it feels almost like that: negative
connotations through and through;
deprivation and suffering. It doesn't have
to be like that if you follow these rules.
No food is forbidden if you eat only when
you're hungry and in moderation.
That's not a diet. That's for life.

If you know you can have more tomorrow, you won't feel deprived today

The diet/binge cycle is vicious in the extreme. Dieters get into that cycle (also known as yo-yo dieting) because they know they are meant to diet 'tomorrow'. If it's forbidden tomorrow, it's logical that you'll stuff it in today while it's still 'allowed'. Whereas if you know you can eat a small amount of your favourite food tomorrow as well, you don't have to binge on it today.

Never tell your host(ess) you're on a diet

Dieting is boring. It's what goody-goodies and spoil-sports do. If you want to sidestep these labels, then don't tell. Once your host(ess) starts saying, 'You don't need to diet' or 'It took me three hours slaving over a hot stove', your resistance will crumble.

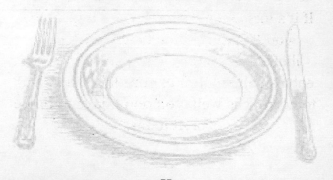

Never allow yourself to become too hungry

That's why the very low-calorie diets don't work in the long run. You go over the top when you can't stand the deprivation any longer. Make sure that you eat when you have a good appetite and don't wait till you're starving. If you wait too long, you won't be able to stop.

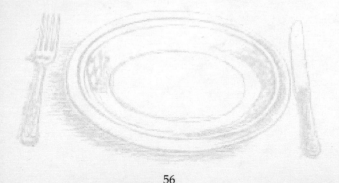

Learn about different kinds of fat

Avoid the bad fat and have a little good fat. We all need some fat in our diet, but make it the right sort. The right sort is fish oil, and oil from seeds, nuts and olives. The wrong sort of oil comes from red meat, dairy products and fried food.

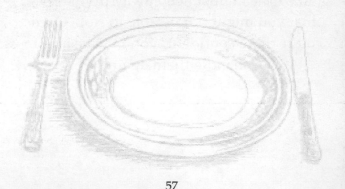

Avoid your true trigger foods

Ideally no food should be forbidden, but you may have certain 'trigger' foods that launch you into binge mode. Peanuts, cheese, chocolates and muesli are common triggers. At the beginning, it may be sensible to cut these foods out altogether for a while. But don't let that stop you choosing other foods you really like instead. Just keep away from those that you might not be able to stop. Once you're more confident, you may be able to handle them again.

Retrain your taste buds

Gradually cut down on processed sugar until you don't want it anymore. No one should be eating much processed sugar, whether they want to lose weight or not. It is empty calories and does nothing for your well-being. The good news is that as you gradually cut down on sweet food, you definitely crave it less. For this reason try and avoid using sweeteners and diet drinks too.

List the disadvantages of being slim

That may seem a strange piece of advice. But if your list is long, then you may find that you're sabotaging your own efforts to lose weight. You might want to do some soul-searching or even seek out a counsellor.

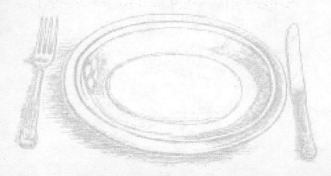

'Low fat' on the label doesn't mean unlimited

You convince yourself that 'low fat' means no calories, so you have two (or ten). Look at the arithmetic of yogurts. A low-fat yogurt is 90 calories and a full-fat yogurt is 130 calories so you'd do better to have one full-fat pot and really enjoy it than two low-fat ones and still hanker after what you really wanted.

Learn about herbs

Herbs aren't just for cranks. They're delicious and they have no calories. Find a book about them and start to experiment – you can use them for flavour instead of sauces. You can even grow them yourself. Chop up chives, spring onions or leeks for a tang. You can make mayonnaise a thing of the past.

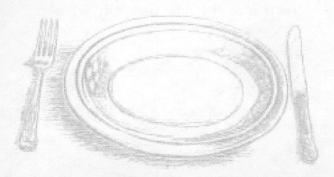

Stand up straight

Standing up straight without any change
to your diet will immediately take half a
stone off you in other people's eyes.
The bonus is that you'll feel better too.
You'll feel energized and ready for
new challenges.

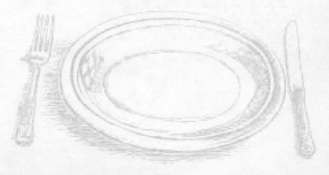

Don't count calories but calories do count

Nothing is more soul-destroying or simply boring than walking around with a little book that lists foods and the calories they contain. Instead, take smaller portions than before. That way you know you're eating less.

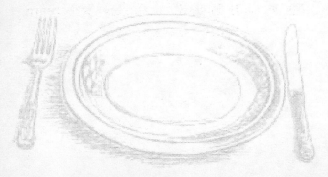

Don't count fat units but fat units do count

Fat units are as dull as calories, but you do have to keep down the fat content of your diet, especially the fats from red meat, yellow cheeses and fried food. Don't count fat units, but make an effort to eat fewer of them. Remember, too, food high in processed sugar is often high in fat, as well. Biscuits, cake and ice cream are all examples.

Use oil sprays if you must 'fry' foods

Oil sprays allow you to use much less oil, but still give you the effect of frying (almost). Get hold of a good non-stick frying-pan.

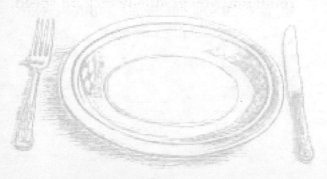

If you skip exercise today, it will be easier to skip it tomorrow

Once you start to stop exercising,
it's difficult to get back into the routine.
Better force yourself to do it every day,
even when you don't feel like it – but take
it at a slower pace on your off days.
You'll find you gradually pick up speed.

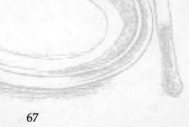

Remember you always have a choice

Knowing that nothing is forbidden gives you a sense of freedom – freedom to choose what it is you really want. If you know you must make a choice, you will think about the pros and cons of each item of food. You are likely to choose wisely if you have the freedom to choose.

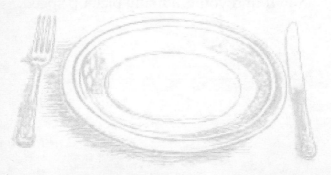

Whoever says that fat people are happy has never been fat

The fat person who is overly jolly is covering up the misery underneath. Nothing could be more true than the saying, 'Inside every fat person is a thin person trying to get out.'

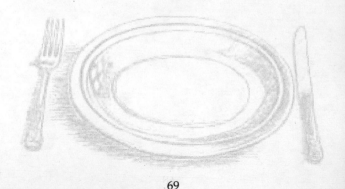

Learn to eat like a naturally slim person

Talk to as many naturally slim people as you can. Most will tell you that they eat when they're hungry – a concept that so many overweight people have completely forgotten. The sooner you adopt it, the sooner you will lose weight for good.

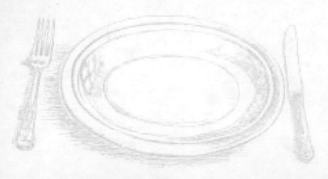

Never walk
if you can run

Although that may be a slight
exaggeration, you could perhaps
realistically say, 'Never walk slowly if
you can walk fast.'

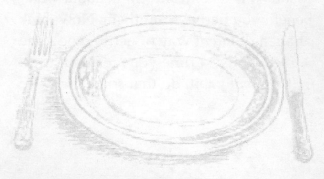

Check how you benefit from a bad habit and find that same benefit elsewhere

Think carefully about what you eat, when you eat it and how you eat it. Can you identify any poor habits? Take those habits one by one and think about what benefit you derive from them. Now think about a different way of getting the same benefit. Next time you are about to indulge that habit, do that something else.

While you eat, always focus on the texture and savour the smell and taste

That way you will slow down and appreciate the food you are eating, and you'll notice you want less.

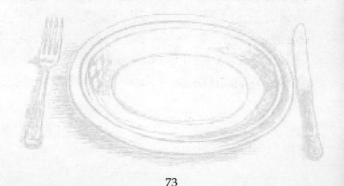

Exercise does not have to be painful to be beneficial

Healthy aerobic exercise that is good for your heart and lungs should be at a pace which still allows you to talk while you're doing it. If you're gasping for breath, slow down.

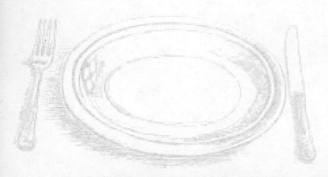

Exercise regularly first thing in the morning

Research shows that those people who exercise first thing in the morning are most likely to keep it up in the long term.

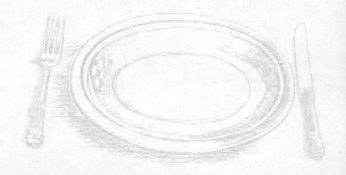

Keep up regular exercise and you'll maintain your weight loss

Research shows that permanent weight loss after conventional dieting is achieved by only a minority of dieters. Those who have kept up an exercise programme once they reach their goal weight are most likely to maintain their weight loss.

Convince yourself that exercise is good for your health

Exercise has been shown to reduce: arthritis, back pain, cancer, diabetes, heart disease, high blood pressure, osteoporosis, incidence of infection, stress, strokes and tension.

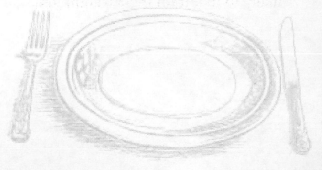

Convince yourself
that exercise
will make you
feel good

Exercise has been shown to improve your posture, your self-esteem, reduce depression and help you sleep better.

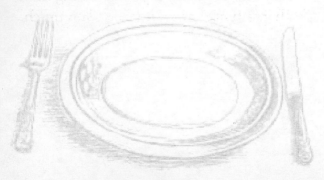

Never take more than a fistful

Portion control is the key to long-term weight management. Some people put on weight because they nibble between meals. That's easy to identify. For those who swear they don't eat between meals, portion size must be the problem. As a very rough guide, if you're eating more than a fistful of an item, it's too much.

Think of your body as a car

You wouldn't put the wrong petrol in
your car, if you wanted it to perform well.
So stop putting poor fuel in your body
if you want a sense of well-being
and energy.

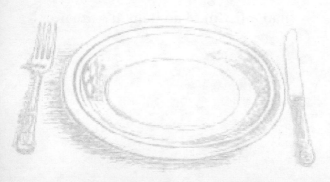

There's no looking back

You will hit difficulties, hitches, plateaux – but just ask yourself honestly whether you want to be back where you started. If you don't move forward, you will move backwards.

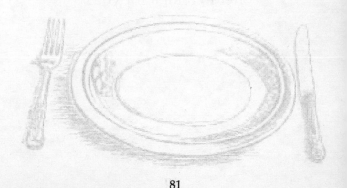

Learn to
sip alcohol

Just as you must learn to nibble food, you must learn to sip alcohol. Alcohol is a double-edged sword. Not only is it full of empty calories but it also makes you care less about your weight-loss goal. You shouldn't have to cut out alcohol, but cut it down by learning to sip. Take a long time to empty your glass so no one will offer to refill it for you.

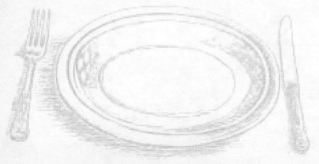

Banish the 'I've blown it' philosophy

If you have a relapse, pick yourself up immediately. Never say, 'I've blown it now so I might as well carry on and start again tomorrow.' That's typical dieters' mentality. You are not on a diet. Just put it behind you and don't eat again until you're hungry.

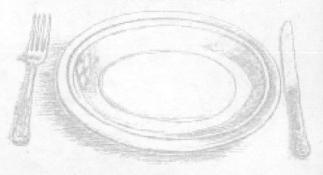

Whatever you do for long enough will become a habit

Remember that there are good habits as well as bad habits. If you eat less sugar for a month, you will get out of the habit and a new sugar-free habit will be born.

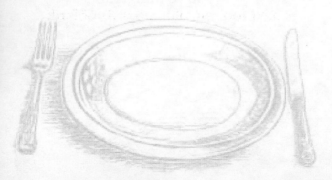

Envisage the weight that you are losing as great lumps of fat

Say you've lost four pounds over the last month. Visualize those four pounds as a lump of lard – four pounds of it. That's a lot. Feel proud that you've got rid of it and you will be motivated to get rid of the next four surplus pounds of lard.

Experiment with beans and lentils

Beans and lentils are very low in fat but full of protein and complex carbohydrates. Choose from black-eyed beans, butter beans, chick peas, haricot beans, kidney beans, lentils and soya beans. If you don't know how to cook them, borrow or buy a vegetarian cookery book.

Reclaim the perfect appetite mechanism that you were born with

Babies are born with a perfect appetite mechanism. They demand food when they're hungry and they stop eating when they're satisfied. We ruin that mechanism by eating for comfort and for reward. Never say to a child, 'I'll give you a biscuit if you stop crying' or 'You can have ice cream if you finish your vegetables.' Attitudes like those caused our problem.

See the funny side of weight loss

Have you ever watched women before
they get weighed in at a weight-loss club?
They go to the toilet, they take off their
shoes, then their belt and lastly their rings.
If you don't laugh you might cry.

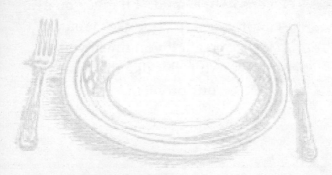

Take a good look at overweight people (don't stare)

Tell yourself you don't want to look like that. It doesn't sound generous or kind, but it is being kind to yourself. Of course, it would be better if we judged others for inner character and not external appearance but none the less…

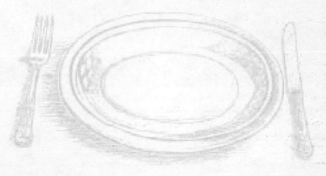

Learn to
be assertive

This is not the same as being aggressive.
'It looks delicious but I couldn't eat
another thing' is an assertive statement.
Remember also that flattery will get you
everywhere. Ask for the recipe.
Ask for a doggy bag.

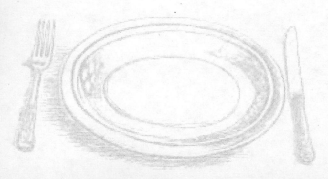

Don't label yourself

You will spoil your efforts if you say things like, 'I'm so greedy' or 'I've got no self-control'. Turn those around and say, 'I can change any behaviour I want.'

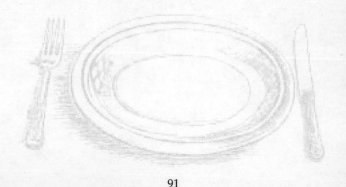

Don't decry your success so far

If you keep saying, 'I've only lost five pounds and I'm bound to put them back on again,' then you will. Instead say, 'I've done well to lose five pounds, and I'm all set to lose the next five.'

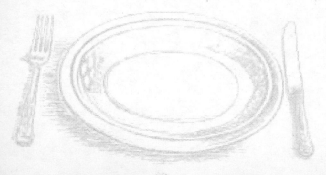

Always
plan ahead

You are learning only to eat when you're hungry, but if your meal times are fixed you must plan to be hungry for them. If you are likely to be hungry before meal time then make sure you have a healthy snack available.

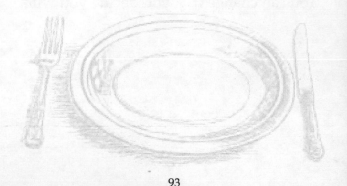

You should love yourself even if you hate the weight

Which is the real you? The large body or the inner person? Start to appreciate your personality and special character. That's what your friends and family appreciate you for. Your body is just the wrapping. You can change it, if you decide you will.

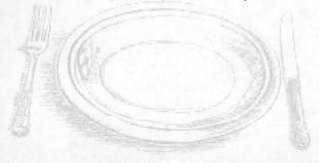

Learn to leave food on your plate

How often do you finish up everything on your plate even though you know you've had enough? Put your napkin down on top of the left-overs to prevent second thoughts. That way the cook can't see what you've left either.

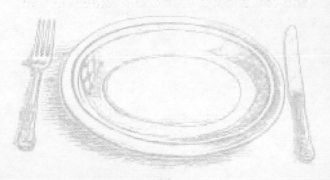

Put on expensive hand cream as you watch TV

This way you'll be less inclined to raid the fridge. It's such a waste to have to wash off all that nice hand cream. You could try lip gloss too as an added precaution.

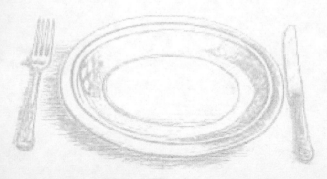

Cut out butter and margarine from sandwiches

Why waste calories on something you can't even taste? You don't taste the butter or margarine under the filling, so just cut it out. But don't put more filling in to make up for it.

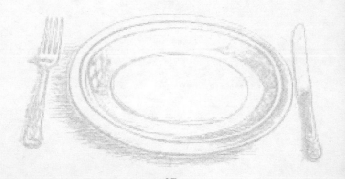

Find alternatives that also taste nice

Never expect an alternative to be the same as the food it's replacing. Consider it a new food. So when you use mustard instead of butter or margarine, enjoy the tang. Don't look for creaminess.

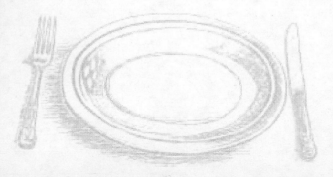

Take it upstairs now

Do you put things on the stairs to take up later? Instead, take them up immediately you think of it. That's probably at least twenty extra flights of stairs in a week – and a tidier house.

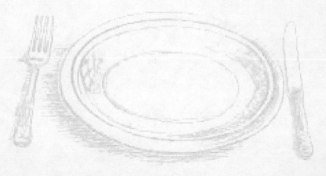

Do stretches to stop you diving into the fridge

As you wait for the kettle or the microwave, are you tempted to open the fridge and straighten the cheese? Do some stretches instead. It's good for your muscles and prevents the nibbling.

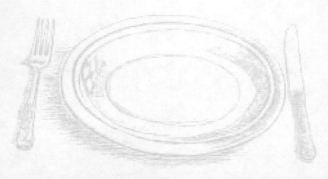

Forget fruit juice and go for the real thing

Eight ounces of orange juice is the equivalent of three whole oranges and has far less fibre. Try eating one whole orange instead and just think how much energy you'll use up when you peel it.

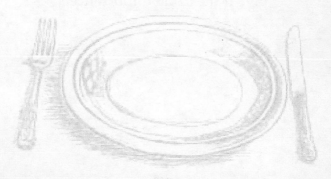

Put exercise
in your diary

What are the most important
commitments that you have in your
diary? Which are the appointments
that you're most reluctant to shift?
Are they business appointments?
Doctor's appointments? Meet-the-teacher
evenings at your child's school?
Now put exercise in your diary and
give it the same importance.

Cook for your family, not for an army

Who eats the left-overs when you cook too much? It's probably you. Could it be that you deliberately cook too much so you can have a private feast in the kitchen? Make a decision to cut back on the cooking.

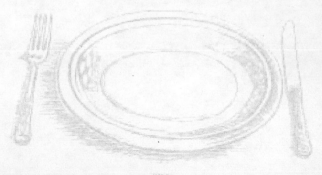

Don't be scared of restaurants

If you enjoy eating out, continue doing so. If eating out precluded staying slim, then all our public figures and film stars would be fat. But don't treat each meal out as your last supper. You can share meals; you can take some home and you can even leave part of them on your plate.

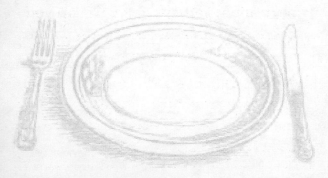

Forget the 'I've paid for it so I have to finish it' attitude

Think of all those things you're paying for when you eat in a restaurant; the food itself is only a small part of what you buy. You're paying for the decor, the atmosphere, the service, for somewhere to be, for the warmth and the lighting, for clean linen, and even for the chef's imagination. Perhaps that will help you realize you're not wasting much if you leave food on your plate.

Ask for
a doggy bag

If the portions are too big, ask the restaurant to wrap up half of it for you to take home as soon as they serve the food. Don't wait till later – there may be nothing left on the plate.

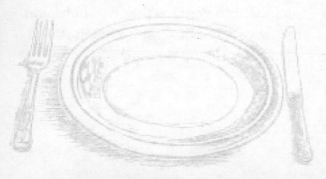

Pretend you're the official taster

At a buffet table, enjoy filling your plate with a spoonful of everything that looks delicious. That way you won't take too much and you won't feel deprived. It will be a treat for your palate. Savour every mouthful and don't go back for more.

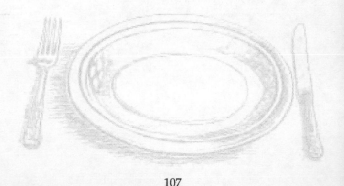

Deliver yourself from temptation

At buffets, help yourself then move far
away from the table and don't go back.
At a restaurant, move the bread rolls to
the other side of the table.

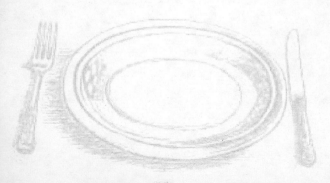

Ask yourself what you're going to go back to

So you're fed up with this new way of eating. Perhaps the scales got stuck this week. You're discouraged. Just think for a moment what awaits you if you go back to your old habits. Self-disgust; a bloated feeling; tight clothes; lethargy; and a whole lot more. Is that what you want?

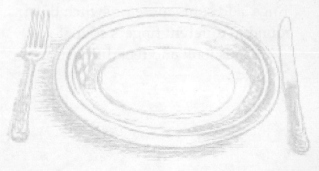

Rings on your fingers...

It's difficult to eat without seeing your fingers. If you've never worn rings, then I suggest you start now – one on each hand. It will feel strange for a while and that's the idea. Let that strangeness remind you of your new habits and the questions you need to ask yourself before you eat. Are you hungry? Are you eating smaller portions more slowly? If you already wear rings, add some more or switch them round to different fingers so that your hands look and feel different.

Start wearing nail varnish – or change your usual colour

Every time you put your hand to your mouth to take a bite and every time you lift a fork to your mouth, you'll see your new-style nails. Let them remind you of your new good habits.

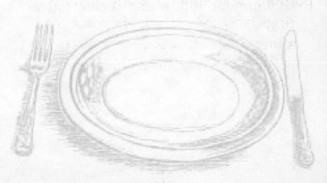

Have a gym at home too

So many people have good intentions. They spend a lot of money joining a gym but just don't have the time to go as often as they'd like. Don't keep saying, 'I'll go.'

Make sure you also have an exercise programme you can do at home for those days when you honestly can't get to the gym. If you can't afford fitness equipment, follow an exercise video.

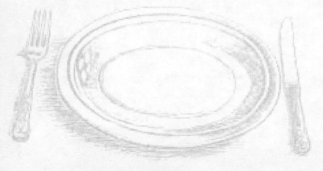

Exercise with your children

Are you a hard-pushed parent with too little time for your children? They will enjoy keeping fit with you and they'll keep you going. It will be good quality time together. It could be an exercise video or skipping or swimming or taking turns on the exercise bike. Use your imagination.

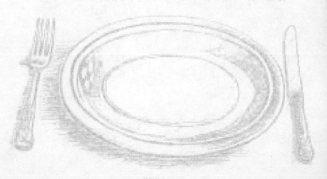

Do the housework in half the time

I'm not suggesting you cut corners.
I mean you should do housework with
gusto. Move faster so that you work up a
good sweat. You'll benefit by saving time
or doing a better job.

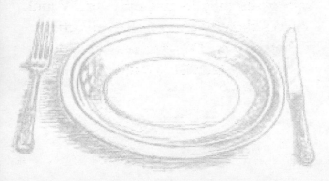

If you can't separate food from television, give up television

So many of us eat mindlessly when we watch television. Whether it's crisps or fruit or even lettuce, if you've just had dinner, you shouldn't be eating. It may seem drastic, but if you've tried unsuccessfully to give up your TV junk food, then fill a week with an activity other than TV. Then reassess your television habits.

Don't eat for a bygone era

If you or your parents grew up during or just after the Second World War, you or they may have learned habits that were good for then but don't work now. Then, when food was rationed, it was important not to waste it. Today we live with over-abundance. Forget the rationing mentality. It's doing you harm.

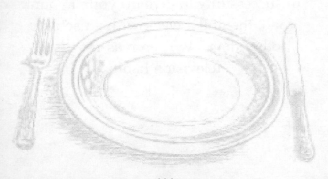

It's important to eat three meals a day

Yes, but are you eating three meals together with six snacks? Do you eat half a meal while you're standing at the fridge preparing it? Do you eat another half-meal when you clear the dishes? Are you eating by the clock instead of by your stomach? Be honest.

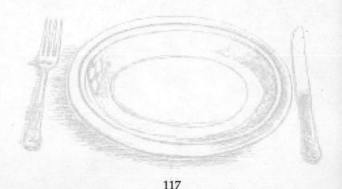

Turn your interest in food into an interest in something else

Choose something interesting, fun, constructive, active . . . Think of all those things you've always wanted to do but you've never had the time. Now you have the time – all the time that you used to spend agonizing over food.

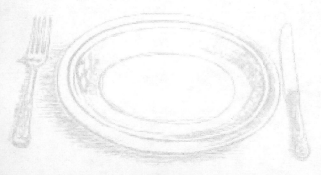

Re-read all these tips regularly

If you do all the things in this book, you will definitely lose weight and keep it off. Keep a different tip uppermost in your mind each day.

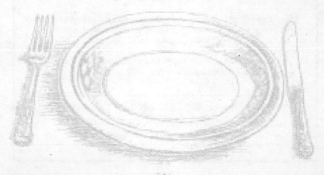